Health
In
Poetry

PETA ZAFIR

Health In Poetry

Book 1

©2021 Peta Zafir

All rights reserved.

No part of this book may be reproduced in any form or by any electronic or mechanical means, including information storage and retrieval systems, without written permission from the author, except in the case of a reviewer, who may quote brief passages embodied in critical articles or in a review.

Trademarked names appear throughout this book. Rather than use a trademark symbol with every occurrence of a trademarked name, names are used in an editorial fashion, with no intention of infringement of the respective owner's trademark.

The information in this book is distributed on an "as is" basis, without warranty. Although every precaution has been taken in the preparation of this work, neither the author nor the publisher shall have any liability to any person or entity with respect to any loss or damage caused or alleged to be caused directly or indirectly by the information contained in this book.

Peta Zafir Publishing
www.petazafir.com

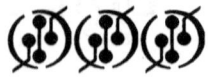

ISBN 978-0-6452140-1-7

Peta Zafir Publishing
www.petazafir.com
Peta Zafir You Tube Channel

BOOKS BY PETA ZAFIR
Health in Poetry Book 1
Health in Poetry Book 2
Book of Sayings Book 1
Book of Sayings Book 2
Book of Sayings Book 3
Book of Sayings Book 4
Scenar For Beginners

All books are available in print and eBook format from:
www.petazafir.com/books

We are now moving into a powerful new time
To work on the baggage, we've been dragging behind
Now it is time for the work to be done
Don't let the past, dim the glow of the sun
Write down your feelings and experience the pain
Then day after day you will feel what you've gained
You have the strength, you lived through the strife
You have the fortitude to regain your new life
No one can stop you, just open up wide
The work that you do will become your clear guide
Out with the old, the sad and tormented
Onward we charge forging paths of contentment
Choose to be happy, let go of the rage
Choose to live now and commence a new page
Each day is a wonder, each hurt we release
Is a moment of joy and a future of peace.

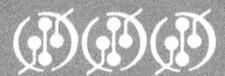

Health in Poetry   Book 1

The Chill has started and cool months have arrived
A little less sun and we fight to survive
We have jobs, and family, sickness and health
And we all seem to focus on the need for more wealth
This stress puts us on an unhealthy road
And the Lack of our sleep just increases the load
If Fun appears fleeting and joys not around
Then you need to follow this plan that I found
Relax and go walking, eat lots of good food
Find friends you can talk to and uplift your mood
Go eat in those places that your love to attend
Take time to reflect so you're able to mend
We all feel at times like the worlds closing in
But change your reactions and learn how to win.

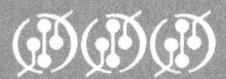

Time travels quickly, days rapidly pass by
Each moment is gone in a blink of an eye
Each morning on waking rejoice in the thought
That you are alive & can achieve what you've sought
Don't leave it a second, a minute or day
Right now is the time that you start on your way
Focus on health, increase energy too
Cut out the sugar, drink water in lieu
Exercise daily, a stroll through the park
Get up off the lounge, watch the morning day start
Don't wait for whenever, don't search for the road
Take a step on the path and lighten your load.

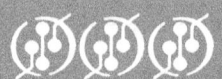

There are many things that affect our lives
So many aspects that can sway our drive
We have to work through the hardships and pain
To clear emotions so contentment can reign
Never stop learning and searching for truth
Never stop clearing your base family root
Never stop letting go of the past
Never stop working and removing your mask
Only then will you know yourself simple & clear
And move into your future releasing all fear.

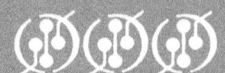

The years pass by full of Hope and good Cheer
Another step closer to the Life you hold dear
Now is the time to commence with your Joy
Now is the time to open up and deploy
Remember be present, live each day complete
Don't wish away time, or drown in defeat
Remember that every day you can Renew
Building the future that is out there for YOU
Start right this second, this minute, this day
Adapt every action and create your own way.

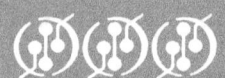

Many people have health conditions
And need to change their life's decisions
Their decreased wellbeing may limit their life
And choices are needed to reduce all their strife
If you are assisting and giving your time
Between Helping and Victim's, a very fine line
You cannot be everything to everyone else
Without losing the part that makes you yourself
Helping is noble and charitable and kind
However, make sure you conserve your own time.

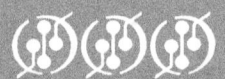

Transform your Future, Extend your Range,
Make a Difference, Achieve the Change,
Act in the Present, Follow your Dreams
Gather your Knowledge, Make up your Team
Make a Plan, Think it Through
Don't Regret, Start Anew
Love Yourself, Find Your Passion
Accept Others, Don't follow the Fashion
Drink Clean Water, Go for a Walk
Eat nourishing Food and Begin a new Sport
Change Today, Don't Hesitate
Believe in the Future; That you can Create.

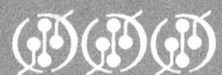

In a flash, each month is finally here
Yet slow down and focus on JOY not your fears
Each day must be started clean and anew
And each daily moment, lived fully and new
Feelings and emotions of the past must be cleared
What matters you need to hold tight and keep near
Walk slowly, keep going, wherever your lead
Never look sideways, you path is ahead.
Always be kind, let your mind and heart grow
Relax, release love and let happiness flow.

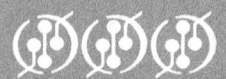

As each month comes, you must watch for signs
The weather changes & you say you're just fine
Maybe this is so and maybe it's not
You need to look inwards and take charge of your lot
When life was given, a path was laid out
Your family, experiences & pain brought in doubt
Remember that you are a one of a kind
No one is you, not in spirit or mind
Realise that now, and discover and learn
To acquire the life that only you earn
Walk to the beat of your personal drum
And find your own rhythm and never succumb.

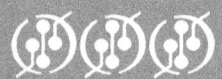

Today is the month that I'm off and away
I am flying to London, the 10th is the day
My son has his 30th birthday this year
And I will be partying with gusto and cheer
Then off to Iceland we depart the next day
And though it is winter, in hot springs we'll stay
Then, into Italia, the Blue Grotto to see
And driving the coast of Amalfi we'll flee
Climb Mt Vesuvius oh what stories I'll tell
Then home again, home again, where I do dwell
I return once again to the work that I do
And there I relate all my stories to you.

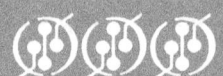

This year is moving so very fast
And Mental Health is here at last
We need to clean and feed our Brain
So all our thoughts will be maintained
Then in old age you can have no fear
Your thinking will remain ever so clear
There are things that you should really know
That many games help the brain to grow
Things to stop and others to take
Begin today it is never too late.

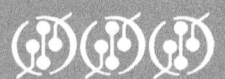

The Time has come for fun this year
So much to do and so much to clear
Now go into action and clean up your act
Exercise, water and increase your good fats
Detox using oils, adding herbs that's the trick
Heavy metals & toxins can make you so sick
Alkalised water removing chlorine
Make sure it's remineralised, taking out the fluorine
Walk on the beach or out on the grass
Breathing fresh air and distressing at last
If something's not right, then you raise up your voice
Remember that happiness is making a choice.

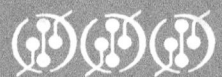

Today is the time we must focus anew
Doing the work to make a breakthrough
Choices today put us on a new road
Happiness, hope and a much lighter load
Make healthy choices and feel so much better
Increase your energy and sleep so much deeper
Go to the toilet and bounce out of bed
Have shiny clear skin and a much clearer head
Clearing the past and letting it go
Finding the path for today's healthy flow
Good choices need to be made don't delay
So come and make sure that you start right today.

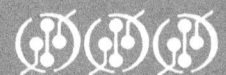

April's arrived and is here with us
She has arrived again without much fuss
The leaves are falling, the weathers cool
The rain is pouring, the trees stand still
We light the torches, and walk the streets
We band together, and talk of their feats
We speak of the Fallen, and remember the last
Of the brave men who fought, and the ANZACS gone past.

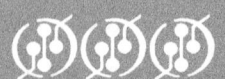

Parts of the year bring temperature change
Shorter days and a lot more rain
Cool breezes and the seas are high
Hot day pass with a welcome sigh
This is the time to take care of your health
Nothing else matters not work or your wealth
Mobility, action and fun in your life
Come from releasing all negative strife
Age is not a factor here
A number need not be attached to fear
Speak, join in and make sure that you laugh
Always make happiness your focus and Path.

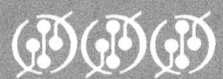

The Path is clear we know where to go
However, our fears start to ebb the flow
Work through your history, and your body will know
That your future is strong and your presence aglow
Today is the day you make the choice
Choose to take charge of your inner source
Let the power within stand up and fight
Don't focus and ponder on all your past plights
Open your heart and never lose sight
Today is the day that you turn on your light.

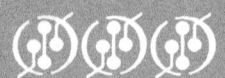

Some months they warn us that winter is near
Start to make plans so you'll have no fear
Build up your strength and start to eat strong
Get ready your body as the days become long
Increase your support and waters a must
As it gets colder warm teas you can trust
Honey and Lemon in water will do
Remember the stomach's your immune system too
Don't wait till later right now you must start
Get moving, and choose to stat living health smart.

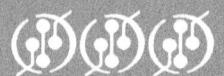

Now is the start of our cold Winter time
Of hot veggie soups with light sprigs of thyme
Bright Fluffy slippers and rugging up tight
Snuggling in doonas and blankets at night
Winter has come with her dark winter coat
The weather is chilly and warm days' remote
Remember that throughout these cold winter days
Support your health and keep sickness away.

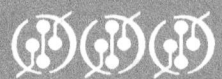

Months pass so quickly and oh what a year
Sometimes blue skies and laughter and cheer
However, the storms can bring floods and the rain
Leaving some people feeling great loss and pain
Whatever happens, what personal plight
There are people who come to shine a new light
Happiness, joy, friendship and time
Show us the strength, we sometimes can't find
When you have sad times and soft flowing tears
Let actions of love, relieve you of fear.

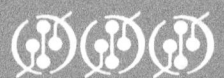

Aging is on us, and increases each year
How do you feel, is your path very clear
Illness and trauma, pain and disease
They limit your movements and give you no ease
Life without Pain is the way it should be
You need to always be moving pain free
You need to be able to turn and bend down
You need to be able to walk and prance round
Pain once you have it does not need to stay
Remember that there is not only one way
Search and ask questions, research all around
There is someone for you, so seek till they're found.

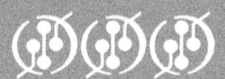

The warmer days have now gone past
And Father Time is moving fast
Half the year has come and gone
And days are darker at the dawn
The sun starts to shade at early noon
And night is lighted by the moon
Exercise is not always done
And our energy suffers from lack of sun
Time to wake the Organs up
Feed and Clean, Reduce the Muck
Spring clean your home and body too
Warm soups and herbal teas for you.

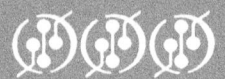

There are some months that bring the cold and the rain
However, within us there is sunshine to gain
Let your time be well spent doing things that you love
Share experiences with others and join a fun club
Remember today will not be forever
When altering your health never say never
Start every day with a small little change
Make some food choices, and start to exchange
Don't be disheartened, your body will help
Look up and walk forward to regain your good health.

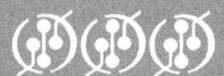

The storms have passed and the cold is here
What a time we have had this year
Changing temperatures, Hot and Cold
Changing patterns of weather untold
There is always a time that we must support health
And sometimes this comes at the cost of our wealth
A requirement of ageing is not to have Pain
Through ageing we also have so much to gain
The wisdom and lessons we walk with today
Allow us to walk in a more youthful Way.

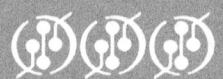

Today is the day, it's time you must start
Renewing your health and supporting your Heart
The arteries and veins need to gently flow
The Heart is the pump and says where to go
Make sure that you eat good nutrition
And add clean water for easy transition
Stop dairy and clean the toxins away
Support your body and start today.

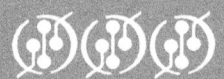

The sun is shining
The skies are clear
The time has come
You can start right here
Take Lots of vegetables
Eat fruit too
And place the focus on
Only You.

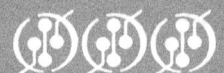

The year will bring a changing time
Of weather, people and love entwined
For some an occasion, a wedding, a joy
Families uniting and times to enjoy
Remember the times that we loved and we laughed
Remember those times that appeared in the past
Start living your happiness every day of your life
You deserve to make choices that lead you from strife
You are unique and are one of a kind
Live your life always with a positive mind.

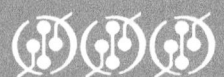

Spring opens up with her colourful glow
And says it's a time to plant & grow
Do simple things that won't take long
That support your health and keep you strong
You don't want illness in your life
You don't want to wait till your health's in strife
Make your choices to guide you through
Then the rest is always up to you
Stick to a plan and follow the lead
Grounding, fresh air and toxin free feed
Have a treatment, get some rest
Bring your health to its Very Best.

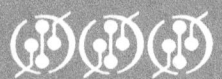

Months keep passing, we focus our time
On our Heart, its health, its strength and rhythm
We centre strongly, on its physical beat
However, its energy may sometimes retreat
If you have been dealing with life's shocks and pain
Our heart starts to shut down and makes us feel drained
Heart break is real and we suffer a lot
We need to talk openly, about what is not
If you've lost a loved one or sickness is here
If the people around you are not close or near
If sadness has started to take over your lives
Let others support you and allow you to thrive
If you're not coping and trying to be strong
Talk it out, feel it and clear what is wrong.

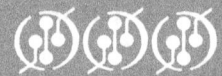

The blanket of winter is lifting aside
The warmth of spring is stretching out wide
The flowers know it is time to grow
And we need to step out and walk, run or go
The body needs moving, the food must be good
The blood needs to circulate, around as it should
The lymph needs some exercise, walk and relax
And your brain needs activity, to remember its facts
Write down your thoughts, keep trouble away
Get up each morning to start the new day.

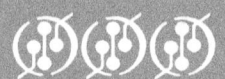

The sun has come the days begun
Make today matter, have a walk or a run
The dawn has cleaned yesterday away
And handed a beginning of a clear new day
Spend some time to feel and write
To clarify your inner fight
Give yourself one day of rest
Pack up emotions and do your best
You walk this path only once in life
Try not to fill it with pain and strife
Give yourself this moment to smile
Feel happiness and joy just for a while
Remember that this too shall pass
Nothing in life will ever last.

Peta Zafir Publishing
www.petazafir.com
Peta Zafir You Tube Channel

BOOKS BY PETA ZAFIR
Health in Poetry Book 1
Health in Poetry Book 2
Book of Sayings Book 1
Book of Sayings Book 2
Book of Sayings Book 3
Book of Sayings Book 4
Scenar For Beginners

All books are available in print and eBook format from:
www.petazafir.com/books

Notes

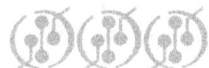

Your Poetry

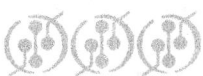

Notes

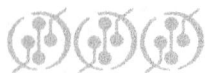

Your Poetry

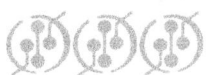

Notes

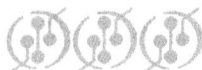

YOUR POETRY

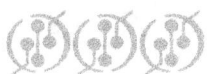

NOTES

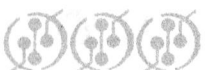

Your Poetry

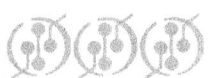

Notes

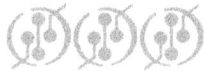

Your Poetry

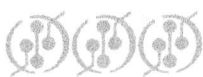

Notes

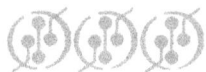

Your Poetry

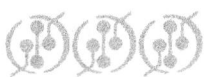

Notes

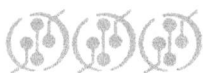

Your Poetry

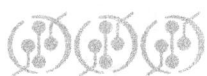

NOTES

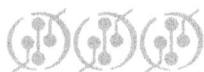

Your Poetry

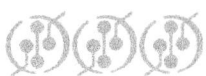

Notes

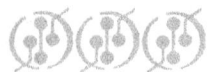

Your Poetry

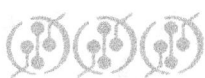

Notes

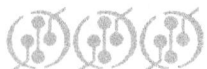

www.ingramcontent.com/pod-product-compliance
Lightning Source LLC
Chambersburg PA
CBHW071837290426
44109CB00017B/1836